CANCER DIET RECIPE FOR KIDS

Nutritious and Kid-Friendly Recipes for Fighting Cancer

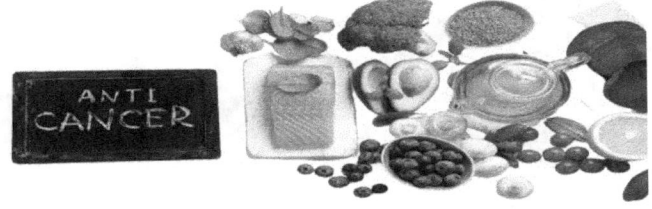

Benjamin Aaron

Copyright © 2022 by Benjamin Aaron.

No part of this publication may be reproduced, distributed, or transmitted in any form or by any means, including photocopying, recording, or other electronic or mechanical methods, without the prior written permission of the copyright holder, except in the case of brief quotations embodied in critical reviews and certain other noncommercial uses permitted by copyright law.

TABLE OF CONTENT

CHAPTER 1 1

INTRODUCTION 1
    CANCER 3
    TYPES OF CANCER AFFECTING CHILDREN 4
    SYMPTOMS OF CANCER IN CHILDREN 6
    DIAGNOSING CANCER 8

CHAPTER 2 10

THE BASICS OF A CANCER DIET FOR KIDS 11
    Foods to include: 13
    Foods to Avoid: 14

CHAPTER 3 15

BENEFITS OF EATING A HEALTHY CANCER DIET 15

CHAPTER 4 20

EASY CANCER DIET RECIPES FOR KIDS 21
BREAKFAST RECIPES *21*
    1. Banana-Blueberry Smoothie Bowl: 21
    2. Peanut Butter and Jelly Overnight Oats: 22
    3. French Toast Sticks: 23
    4. Egg and Cheese Quesadillas: 24
    5. Avocado Toast: 24
    6. Yogurt Parfait: 25
    7. Apple Cinnamon Pancakes: 25
    8. Breakfast Burritos: 26
    9. Oatmeal with Berries and Nuts: 27
    10. Breakfast Sandwich: 27

LUNCH RECIPES *28*
    7. Quesadillas 32
    10. Peanut Butter and Banana Sandwich 34

DINNER RECIPES 34
 1. Macaroni and Cheese 34
SNACK RECIPES 42
DESSERT RECIPES 48

CHAPTER 5 56

MEAL PLANNING 57

DAY 1 59
 BREAKFAST: 59
 LUNCH: 60
 DINNER: 61

DAY 2 63
 BREAKFAST: 63
 LUNCH: 64
 DINNER: 65

DAY 3 67
 BREAKFAST: 67
 LUNCH: 68
 DINNER: 69

DAY 4 70
 BREAKFAST: 70
 LUNCH: 71
 DINNER: 73

DAY 5 74
 BREAKFAST: 74
 LUNCH: 75
 DINNER: 76

DAY 6 77
 BREAKFAST: 77
 LUNCH: 78
 DINNER: 80

DAY 7 81
 BREAKFAST: 81

LUNCH: 82
DINNER: 83
CHAPTER 5 86
TIPS FOR ENCOURAGING KIDS TO EAT HEALTHY 87
LIFESTYLE CHANGES TO CONSIDER 90
CONCLUSION 93

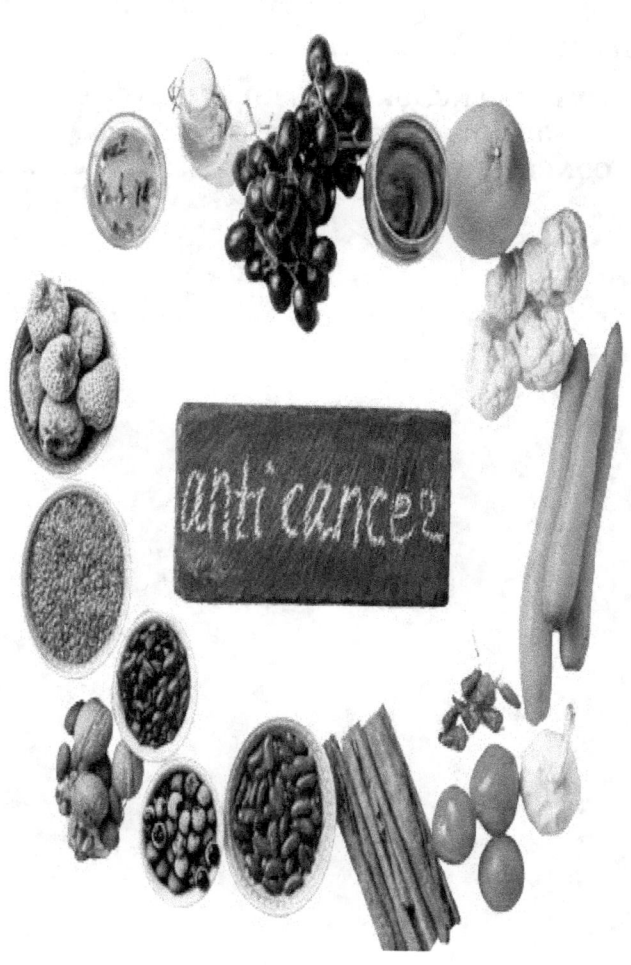

CHAPTER 1

INTRODUCTION

Janet was the single mother of a 4-year-old boy who was diagnosed with cancer. She was devastated and desperate to do anything to help her son fight this deadly disease.

One day, while searching for a solution, she stumbled upon a book entitled "Cancer Diet Recipe for Kids." She read the book from cover to cover and was amazed at the amount of information it contained about diet and nutrition for kids battling cancer. She quickly realized that the right diet and nutrition were key to helping her son battle cancer.

With a newfound hope, Janet began to implement the diet and nutrition plan outlined in the book. She cooked meals rich in vitamins, minerals, and antioxidants while avoiding processed foods and sugar. She also started giving her son supplements that were specifically designed for cancer patients.

Within a few months, Janet noticed a remarkable improvement in her son's health. His cancer was slowly beginning to regress, and he was becoming stronger every day. Janet was so relieved and thankful that she decided to continue following the diet and nutrition guidelines outlined in the book.

Fast forward to today, and Janet's son is now 8 years old and cancer-free. She is so proud of her son and deeply grateful for the book that helped her fight her son's cancer. To this day, she continues to follow the diet and nutrition plan outlined in the book, ensuring that her son remains healthy and cancer-free.

Janet's story is a reminder that with the right diet and nutrition plan; even the most daunting health challenges can be overcomed.

A kid's cancer diagnosis can come as a terrible shock to the parents and other family members who care for that youngster. When cancer strikes, the family is immediately in difficulty. How the family and loved ones navigate and manage these trying times is very important. Having the requisite knowledge can bring calmness and stability in health to both the child and his or her parents. As a result, we present to you a comprehensive guide with a well-detailed, holistic, and kid-friendly approach to managing and preventing cancer in children. You'll discover in this book that good nutrition is crucial to kids' overall health, but it's even more crucial for kids who are undergoing cancer treatment. This book will assist you in understanding how cancer and its treatment may influence your kid as well as their dietary needs. To assist you in making sure your child is receiving the nutrients they require, we also provide tips and kid-friendly recipes.

CANCER

Cancer is a term used to describe a group of diseases

characterized by abnormal and uncontrolled cell growth. Children are not exempt from the effects of cancer. After accidents, cancer is the second most common cause of mortality in children.

TYPES OF CANCER AFFECTING CHILDREN

The most common types of cancer that affect children include leukemia, brain tumors, lymphoma, rhabdomyosarcoma, neuroblastoma, and wilms tumor.

LEUKEMIA: A kind of cancer of the blood and bone marrow is called leukemia. It affects the production of white blood cells, which help the body fight infection. In children, the most common type is acute lymphoblastic leukemia (ALL), which is an aggressive form of the disease that can quickly spread throughout the body.

BRAIN TUMORS: Brain tumors can occur in children of any age. They are generally divided into two categories: malignant and benign. While benign tumors are not carcinogenic, malignant ones are. Depending on the type and location, brain tumors can cause a wide range of symptoms, such as headaches, vision problems, balance issues, and seizures.

LYMPHOMA: Lymphoma is a type of cancer that affects the lymphatic system, which is part of the immune system. In children, the most common type of lymphoma is non-Hodgkin's lymphoma. Symptoms of lymphoma can include swollen lymph nodes, fever, night sweats, and fatigue.

RHABDOMYOSARCOMA: Rhabdomyosarcoma is a rare type of cancer that affects the muscles. It is the most common type of soft tissue cancer in children and adolescents. Symptoms of rhabdomyosarcoma include swelling or a lump in the affected area, pain, and difficulty moving.

NEUROBLASTOMA: A kind of cancer that damages nerve cells is called neuroblastoma. Infants and small children are most commonly affected. Symptoms of neuroblastoma can include abdominal pain, a lump in the abdomen, and bone pain.

WILMS TUMOR: kidney cancer of the Wilms tumor kind mostly affects young people. It is the most common type of kidney cancer in children and the most common type of childhood cancer overall. Symptoms of a Wilms tumor can include abdominal pain, a lump in the abdomen, and blood in the urine.

These types of cancers represent more than half of all childhood cancer cases. The primary risk factor for childhood cancer is exposure to radiation, although there are many other potential causes. These include exposure to certain chemicals and viruses, genetic factors, and a history of certain medical conditions.

SYMPTOMS OF CANCER IN CHILDREN

Cancer in children can present with various symptoms, depending on the type and location of the tumor. Common symptoms may include:

- Unexpected weight loss or appetite loss
- Unexplained fever or night sweats
- Unexplained pain or swelling in any part of the body
- Constant fatigue
- Unexplained paleness or lack of energy
- Unexplained bruising or bleeding
- A palpable bulge or bump under the skin
- Difficulty breathing or persistent cough
- Recurring infections
- Swelling of lymph nodes
- Headaches, vomiting, and/or seizures (in some cases)

It is important to note that some of these symptoms can be attributed to other illnesses, so it is essential to consult a doctor if any of these symptoms are observed. In addition, some types of cancer may not present any symptoms at all, so it is important to be aware of the risk factors associated with each type of cancer and to get regular check-ups to monitor for any changes.

DIAGNOSING CANCER

Cancer in children is a rare but very serious condition. Diagnosing cancer in children can be a complicated process, as there are many different types of cancer and many different signs and symptoms that can be associated with it. Generally, the diagnosis of cancer in children involves a combination of physical exams, imaging tests, laboratory tests, and biopsies.

Physical exams are usually the first step in the diagnosis of cancer in children. During this exam, the doctor will check the child's physical appearance, look for any signs of the disease, including lumps, bumps, or swelling, and take a detailed medical history. Imaging tests such as X-rays, CT scans, and MRI scans may be used to help diagnose cancer in children. These scans provide detailed images of the inside of the body and can help identify any abnormalities that may be indicative of cancer.

Laboratory tests are also used to help diagnose cancer in children. These tests involve taking a sample of the child's blood, urine, or other body fluid and analyzing it for any abnormalities that may indicate the presence of cancer. In some cases, a sample of the tumor may also be taken for further analysis.

Finally, a biopsy may be used to diagnose cancer in children. During a biopsy, a small piece of tissue is taken from the tumor and examined under a microscope. This can help confirm the presence of cancer and determine the type of cancer.

The diagnosis of cancer in children is a complicated process that involves a combination of physical exams, imaging tests, laboratory tests, and biopsies. It is important to speak to a doctor if you have any concerns about cancer in your child.

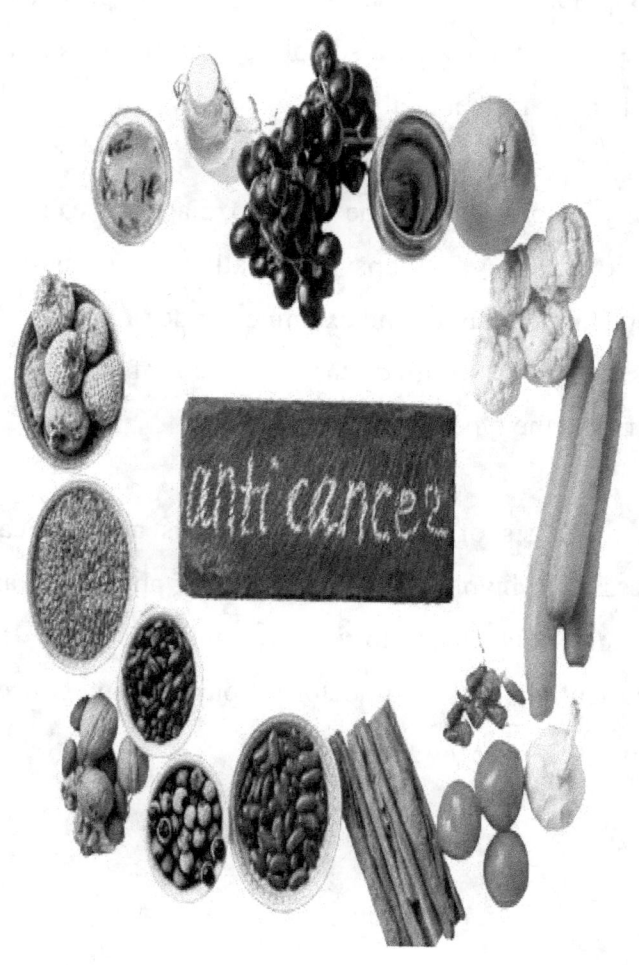

CHAPTER 2

THE BASICS OF A CANCER DIET FOR KIDS

Nutritional needs for children with cancer vary depending on the type of cancer, the treatment, and the individual child. Generally, children with cancer need to meet the same nutritional needs as other children their age. They will likely need a balanced diet that includes a variety of foods from all food groups. A cancer diet for kids is important because the food they eat can help their bodies fight cancer and manage the side effects of treatment. It can also help them maintain a healthy weight, which is important for their overall health and well-being.

The basics of a cancer diet for kids include eating a variety of nutrient-rich, whole foods. This means choosing plenty of fruits, vegetables, lean protein, whole grains, and healthy fats. It also means avoiding highly processed, sugary, and refined foods. Fruits and vegetables are important because they are packed with vitamins, minerals, antioxidants, and fiber. Eating a wide variety of colors and types of fruits and vegetables will ensure that your child is getting the most nutrition from their food.

Lean proteins like fish, poultry, tofu, and beans are important for kids who have cancer. They provide essential amino acids that help the body heal and rebuild. Whole grains are also important because they provide complex carbohydrates that give kids energy throughout the day. Whole-grain bread, pasta, and cereals are all good sources of complex carbohydrates.

Healthy fats like nuts, seeds, and avocados are good sources of energy and essential fatty acids. They can help kids feel satisfied and full after meals. It is important to limit sugary and processed foods, as they can cause inflammation in the body and be difficult to digest. These types of foods are also often high in calories and low in nutrients.

Finally, it is important to stay hydrated. Water is essential for eliminating toxins from the body, helping digestion, and maintaining a healthy weight. By following these basic dietary guidelines, parents can help their children get the nutrition they need to fight cancer and stay healthy.

When planning a nutritional chart for your kid, the following precepts below are noteworthy.

Foods to include:

- High-fiber foods such as whole grains, fruits, vegetables, and legumes
- Lean proteins including tofu, fish, chicken, and eggs
- Wholesome fats from avocados, almonds, and seeds
- Dairy foods such as yogurt and cheese
- Unsweetened beverages such as water, herbal tea, and unsweetened almond milk

Foods to Avoid:

- Added sugars and sweeteners
- Processed and refined foods
- High-sodium foods
- Deep-fried and high-fat foods
- Alcohol and caffeine
- Raw meat and fish
- Artificial colors and flavors
- Foods high in preservatives and additives

It is also important to work with a healthcare professional to determine the best nutrition plan for your child.

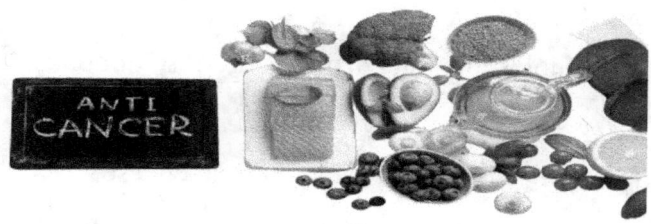

CHAPTER 3

BENEFITS OF EATING A HEALTHY CANCER DIET

When a kid has cancer, proper diet is crucial. However, childhood cancer and its side effects can have an impact on a child's appetite, level of energy, tolerance for particular meals, and nutritional uptake. Children who must stay in the hospital and those who have illnesses and fever should be especially aware of this.

Making sure kids consume the correct foods before, during, and after cancer treatment may benefit them in the following ways:

1. **Boosts the immune system**

A healthy cancer diet should be rich in antioxidants, vitamins, minerals, and other nutrients needed to enhance the immune system, allowing the body to function optimally and fight off infection.

2. Reduces fatigue

A healthy cancer diet helps to reduce fatigue, which is a common side effect of cancer treatments. Eating foods that are high in protein, carbohydrates, and essential fatty acids can provide the body with the energy needed to stay active and reduce fatigue.

3. Enhances healing

Proper nutrition can help reduce inflammation and increase healing, which is necessary for cancer patients. Eating foods full of antioxidants can help reduce oxidative stress, which can lead to cell damage.

4. Improves quality of life

A healthy cancer diet can provide vital nutrients to the body and help a child feel better. Eating a variety of healthy foods can help to improve a child's quality of life, energy levels, and overall well-being.

5. Improves body composition

A healthy cancer diet can help to improve body composition and muscle mass, which can be important in helping to reduce the risk of secondary health complications. Eating a variety of healthy foods can also help reduce the risk of metabolic syndrome and type 2-diabetes.

6. Reduces toxicity

A healthy cancer diet can help to reduce the risk of toxicity associated with chemotherapy, radiation, and other cancer therapies. Eating foods that are rich in antioxidants can help reduce the risk of oxidative damage caused by cancer treatments.

7. Improves mental health

A healthy cancer diet can help to improve mental health and reduce the risk of depression and anxiety. Eating a balanced diet that is full of healthy fats and nutrients can help to improve mood, reduce stress, and increase energy levels.

8. Decreases cancer risk

A healthy cancer diet can help reduce the risk of developing cancer in the future. Eating a variety of nutrient-rich foods may help to reduce the risk of cancer-causing agents, such as free radicals, accumulating in the body.

9. Improves digestion

A healthy cancer diet can help improve digestion, which is important for cancer patients. Eating foods that are high in fiber can help to reduce constipation and other digestive issues associated with cancer treatments.

10. Enhances nutrition

A healthy cancer diet can help to ensure that a child is receiving the essential nutrients needed to stay healthy. Eating a variety of nutrient-rich foods can help reduce the risk of nutrient deficiencies, which can be common in cancer patients.

Maintaining normal growth and development is a major goal of diet and physical exercise for kids with cancer.

Both during and after cancer treatment, this is crucial. Additionally, studies have shown that childhood cancer survivors are more prone than non-survivors to get second malignancies, heart disease, and insulin resistance in their younger years. Early instruction in appropriate eating practices can help children avoid or postpone the development of chronic health disorders later in life.

Children who start and maintain regular exercise also have a decreased chance of dying and a lower probability of their cancer returning.

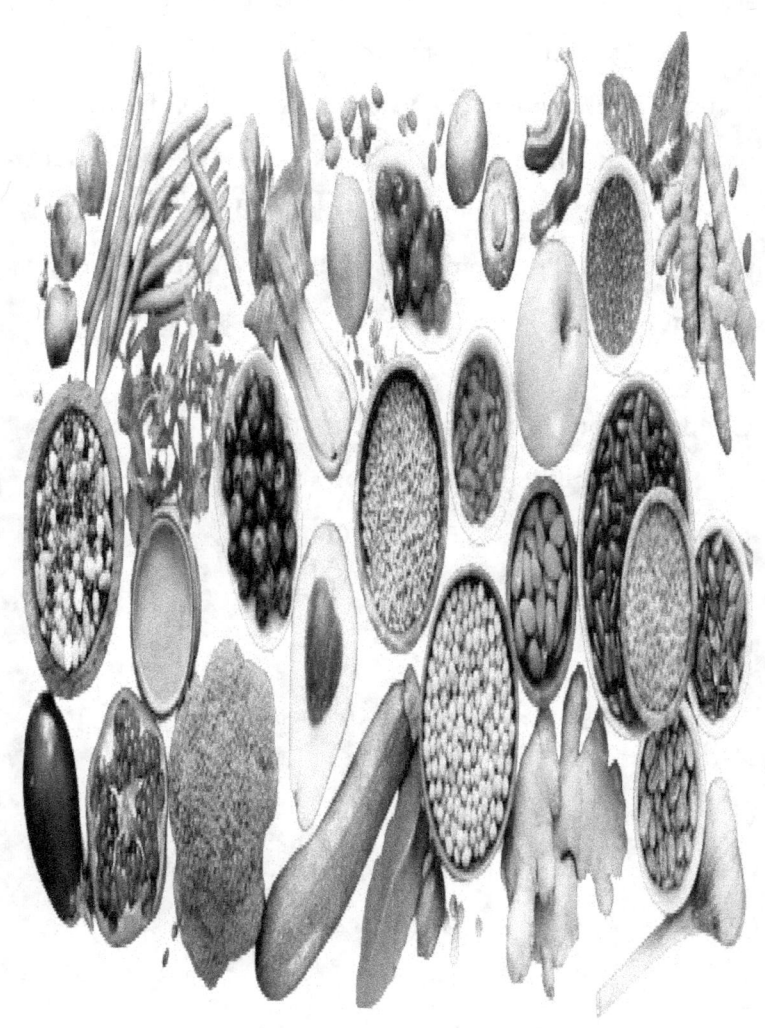

CHAPTER 4

EASY CANCER DIET RECIPES FOR KIDS

Kid-friendly cancer diet recipes are those that are tailored to provide the nutrition needed to support a child's body during cancer treatment, while also being enjoyable to eat. These recipes use fresh, whole ingredients, including fruits and vegetables, lean proteins, and whole grains, to provide the vitamins, minerals, and antioxidants that are essential for healthy growth and development. Meals are also designed to be easy to prepare and appealing to a child's taste buds, making them more likely to be eaten. Examples of kid-friendly cancer diet recipes include:

BREAKFAST RECIPES

1. **Banana-Blueberry Smoothie Bowl:**

Prep Time: 5 minutes

Ingredients:

- 1 frozen banana
- 1/2 cup frozen blueberries
- 1/2 cup plain yogurt
- 2 tablespoons honey
- 1/4 cup granola

Preparation Instructions: In a blender, combine the banana, blueberries, yogurt, and honey. Blend until smooth. Pour the smoothie into a bowl and top with the granola. Enjoy!

2. **Peanut Butter and Jelly Overnight Oats:**

Prep Time: 10 minutes

Ingredients:

- 1/2 cup rolled oats
- 1/2 cup almond milk
- 1 tablespoon peanut butter
- 1 tablespoon chia seeds
- 1/2 teaspoon cinnamon
- 1/2 teaspoon vanilla extract, and
- 2 tablespoons jelly

Preparation Instructions: In a bowl, combine the oats, almond milk, peanut butter, chia seeds, cinnamon, and vanilla extract. Mix until everything is combined. Pour the oats into a Mason jar and top with the jelly. Refrigerate overnight. Serve cold. Enjoy!

3. French Toast Sticks:

Prep Time: 10 minutes
Ingredients:

    2 eggs

    2 tablespoons milk

    1 teaspoon cinnamon

    1/4 teaspoon nutmeg

    4 slices of bread

    2 tablespoons butter

Preparation Instructions: In a shallow bowl, whisk together the eggs, milk, cinnamon, and nutmeg. The butter should be melted in a large pan over medium heat. Bread slices should be dipped into the egg mixture and coated on both sides. Place the slices into the skillet and cook for 3–4 minutes per side or until golden brown. Cut into strips and serve. Enjoy!

4. **Egg and Cheese Quesadillas:**

Prep Time: 10 minutes;

Ingredients:

    4 tortillas

    4 eggs

    1 cup shredded cheese

    1/4 cup milk

    2 tablespoons butter

Preparation Instructions: In a medium bowl, whisk together the eggs, milk, and cheese. In a large pan set over medium heat, melt the butter. Place a tortilla in the skillet and spread 1/4 of the egg mixture on top. Place a second tortilla on top and cook for 3–4 minutes per side or until golden brown and the eggs are cooked through. Cut into wedges and serve. Enjoy!

5. **Avocado Toast:**

Prep time: 5 minutes

Ingredients:

    2 slices of bread

    1 avocado

1/2 teaspoon garlic powder

1/4 teaspoon salt

Preparation Instructions: Toast the bread slices. In a bowl, mash the avocado. Spread the mashed avocado on the toasted bread slices and sprinkle with the garlic powder and salt. Enjoy!

6. Yogurt Parfait:

Prep time: 5 minutes

Ingredients:

1/2 cup plain yogurt

1/4 cup granola

1/4 cup berries

Preparation Instructions: In a bowl, layer the yogurt, granola, and berries. Enjoy!

7. Apple Cinnamon Pancakes:

Prep Time: 10 minutes

Ingredients:

1 cup all-purpose flour,

2 teaspoons baking powder

1 teaspoon cinnamon

1/2 teaspoon salt,

1 cup milk

1 egg

2 tablespoons butter, and

One peeled and diced apple

Preparation Instructions: In a bowl, whisk together the flour, baking powder, cinnamon, and salt. Mix the milk, egg, and butter in a separate basin. After adding the liquid ingredients, mix the dry ingredients just until combined. Fold in the diced apples. Heat a large skillet over medium heat and melt a tablespoon of butter. Pour 1/4 cup of batter into the skillet and cook for 2-3 minutes per side or until golden brown. Serve with maple syrup. Enjoy!

8. **Breakfast Burritos:**

Prep Time: 10 minutes

Ingredients:

4 eggs

1/2 cup black beans

1/2 cup diced bell pepper

1/4 cup shredded cheese

4 tortillas

2 tablespoons olive oil

Preparation Instructions: Heat a large skillet over medium heat and add the olive oil. Add the eggs, black beans, bell pepper, and cheese to the skillet and scramble until the eggs are cooked through. Place the scramble into the tortillas and wrap up. Enjoy!

9. Oatmeal with Berries and Nuts:

Prep Time: 5 minutes

Ingredients:

1 cup rolled oats

1 cup almond milk

1/4 cup berries

2 tablespoons chopped nuts

Preparation Instructions: In a saucepan, combine the oats, almond milk, berries, and nuts. Cook over medium heat for five minutes or until the oats are cooked through. Serve warm. Enjoy!

10. Breakfast Sandwich:

Prep Time: 5 minutes

Ingredients:
- 2 slices of bread
- 1 egg
- 2 slices of cheese
- 2 slices of ham

Preparation Instructions: Heat a large skillet over medium heat and add the egg. Cook for two to three minutes or until the egg is cooked through. Build the sandwich with the bread, egg, cheese, and ham. Enjoy!

LUNCH RECIPES

1. Turkey and Cheese Wraps

Prep Time: 10 minutes

Ingredients:
- 2 whole wheat tortillas
- 2 slices of turkey
- 2 slices of cheese
- 1 tablespoon of mayonnaise
- Lettuce and tomato

Preparation: Spread mayonnaise on the tortillas, then layer the turkey and cheese. Top with lettuce and tomato. Roll up the wraps and cut them in half.

2. Egg Salad Sandwich

Prep Time: 10 minutes

Ingredients:

    4 boiled eggs

    2 tablespoons of mayonnaise

    2 slices of whole wheat bread,

    Lettuce and tomato

Preparation: Mash the eggs with a fork and stir in the mayonnaise. Spread the egg salad on the bread and top with lettuce and tomato.

3. Grilled Cheese Sandwich

Prep Time: 10 minutes

Ingredients:

    2 slices of whole wheat bread

    2 slices of cheese

    1 tablespoon of butter

Preparation: Heat a skillet over medium heat. Spread the butter on one side of each slice of bread and place one slice of bread, butter side down, in the skillet. Place the cheese on top of the bread, then add the second slice of bread with the butter side up. Grill each side of the sandwich until the cheese is melted and the bread is golden brown.

4. Stir Fry - Prep Time:

Prep Time : 10 minutes
Ingredients:

    1 cup cooked brown rice

    1 tablespoon olive oil

    1/2 cup diced vegetables (such as bell peppers, carrots, and broccoli)

    1/4 cup cooked chicken

    1 tablespoon soy sauce

Preparation: Heat the olive oil in a large skillet over medium heat. Add the vegetables and cook for 5 minutes, stirring occasionally. Add the chicken and cook for an additional 2 minutes. Add the cooked rice and soy sauce, and stir to combine. Cook for an additional 3 minutes, stirring occasionally.

5. Macaroni and Cheese

Prep Time: 10 minutes

Ingredients:

    1 cup uncooked macaroni

    2 tablespoons butter

    2 tablespoons flour

    1 cup milk, and

    1/2 cup shredded cheese

Preparation: Bring a pot of water to a boil and cook the macaroni according to the package directions. Melt the butter in a pot while it's still warm. Add the flour and stir until combined. Add the milk gradually while whisking, then heat until thickened. Remove from the heat and stir in the cheese until melted. Return the macaroni to the saucepan after draining. After adding the cheese sauce, mix the macaroni with it.

6. Chicken Salad

Prep Time: 10 minutes

Ingredients:

    1/2 cup cooked chicken

    1/4 cup diced celery

    1/4 cup diced apples

1/4 cup mayonnaise

1 tablespoon lemon juice

Lettuce and tomato

Preparation: In a medium bowl, combine the chicken, celery, apples, mayonnaise, and lemon juice. Mix until well combined. Serve on a bed of lettuce and tomatoes.

7. Quesadillas

Prep Time: 10 minutes

Ingredients:

2 whole wheat tortillas

1/4 cup black beans

1/4 cup corn

1/4 cup shredded cheese

1 tablespoon olive oil

Preparation: Over medium heat, warm the olive oil in a skillet. Place one tortilla in the skillet and top with the beans, corn, and cheese. Place the second tortilla on top. Cook for 2-3 minutes, flipping once, until the cheese is melted and the tortillas are golden brown. Cut into wedges and serve.

8. Tuna Salad - Prep Time:

Prep Time : 10 minutes

Ingredients:

    1 can tuna

    1/4 cup diced celery

    1/4 cup diced apples

    2 tablespoons mayonnaise

    Lettuce and tomato

Preparation: In a medium bowl, combine the tuna, celery, apples, and mayonnaise. Mix until well combined. Serve on a bed of lettuce and tomatoes.

9. Mini Pizzas

Prep Time: 10 Minutes

Ingredients:

    2 English muffins

    1/4 cup pizza sauce,

    1/4 cup shredded cheese

    1/4 cup diced vegetables (such as bell peppers, onions, and mushrooms)

Preparation: Preheat the oven to 350°F. Split the English muffins in half and spread the pizza sauce on each half. Top with the cheese and vegetables. Place on a baking sheet and bake for 10 minutes, or until the cheese is melted and the muffins are golden brown.

10. Peanut Butter and Banana Sandwich

Prep Time: 10 minutes –

Ingredients:

    2 slices of whole wheat bread

    2 tablespoons peanut butter

    1 banana, sliced

Preparation: Spread the peanut butter on the bread. Top with the sliced banana. Piece in half the top slice of bread and the bottom slice.

DINNER RECIPES

1. Macaroni and Cheese

Prep Time: 10 minutes

Ingredients

    2 cups macaroni

2 tablespoons Butter

2 tablespoons all-purpose flour

1 teaspoon salt

1/4 teaspoon ground black pepper

2 cups milk

1 cup grated cheddar cheese

Preparation Instructions: Bring a large pot of lightly salted water to a boil. Add macaroni and cook for 8 to 10 minutes, until al dente. Drain. In a medium saucepan, melt the butter over medium heat. Stir in the flour, salt, and pepper until blended. Pour in the milk, stirring constantly until the mixture thickens. Add the cheese and stir until melted. Add the cooked macaroni and stir to coat.

2. Grilled Cheese and Tomato Soup

Prep Time: 10 minutes

Ingredients:

    4 slices of bread

    2 tablespoons Butter

    4 slices of cheese

    2 cans tomato soup

Preparation Instructions: Pre-heat a large skillet over low heat. Each slice of bread should have butter on one side. Butter side down, place two pieces of bread in the skillet. Each piece of bread should have a slice of cheese on it. Butter-side up, add the remaining slices of bread on top. After lightly browning one side, turn the food over and continue cooking. Meanwhile, heat the tomato soup in a medium saucepan over medium heat. Serve the tomato soup and the grilled cheese sandwiches.

3. Baked Chicken Fingers

Prep Time: 15 minutes

Ingredients:

2 boneless, skinless chicken breasts

1 cup bread crumbs

1 teaspoon garlic powder

1 teaspoon onion powder

1/2 teaspoon salt

1/4 teaspoon black pepper

1 egg, 2 tablespoons olive oil

Preparation Instructions: Pre-heat the oven to 400°F. Cut the chicken breasts into strips. In a shallow bowl, mix together the bread crumbs, garlic powder, onion powder, salt, and pepper. Beat the egg in a separate shallow bowl. Dip each chicken strip into the egg, then into the bread crumb mixture. Place the strips on a baking sheet. Drizzle with olive oil. Bake for 12-15 minutes, until cooked through and golden brown.

4. Fish Sticks and French Fries

Prep Time: 10 minutes

Ingredients:

    1 package of frozen fish sticks

    1 package of frozen french fries

Preparation Instructions: Pre-heat the oven to 425°F. Place the fish sticks on a baking sheet. Bake for 10 minutes, until cooked through. Meanwhile, place the french fries on a separate baking sheet. Bake for 10-15 minutes, until golden brown and crispy. Serve the fish sticks with the french fries.

5. Pizza Quesadillas

Prep Time: 10 minutes

Ingredients:

4 flour tortillas

1 cup shredded mozzarella cheese

1/2 cup pizza sauce

1/2 cup diced pepperoni

Preparation Instructions: Preheat a large skillet over medium heat. Place one tortilla in the pan and sprinkle with 1/4 of the cheese. Top with 1/4 of the pizza sauce and 1/4 of the pepperoni. Place a second tortilla on top. Cook until the cheese is melted for about 1-2 minute. Flip the quesadilla and cook for 1-2 minutes more, until the cheese is melted and the tortillas are golden brown. Repeat with the remaining tortillas. Cut the quesadillas into wedges and serve.

6. Baked Potato Skins

Prep Time: 10 minutes

Ingredients

4 large potatoes,

1/2 cup shredded cheddar cheese

1/4 cup bacon bits

2 tablespoons Butter

1/4 cup sour cream

Preparation Instructions: Pre-heat the oven to 350°F. Scrub and rinse the potatoes. Pierce each potato several times with a fork and bake for 45 minutes, until cooked through. Allow it to cool a little after removing it from the oven. Cut each potato in half lengthwise and scoop out the insides, leaving a thin layer of potato attached to the skins. Place the skins on a baking sheet and top each with 1/4 cup cheese, 1 tablespoon bacon bits, and 1/2 tablespoon butter. Bake for 10 minutes, until the cheese is melted and the skins are golden brown. Serve with sour cream.

7. Vegetable Stir-Fry

Prep Time: 10 minutes

Ingredients:

    1 tablespoon oil
    1/2 cup diced onion
    1 cup diced carrots
    1 cup diced bell peppers
    1 cup broccoli florets
    1/4 cup soy sauce

Preparation Instructions: Heat the oil in a large skillet over medium heat. Cook for 1-2 minute after adding onions. Add the carrots, bell peppers, and broccoli and cook for 5 minutes, stirring occasionally. Add the soy sauce and cook for 2-3 minutes, until the vegetables are tender. Serve.

8. Baked Beans and Hot Dogs

Prep Time: 10 minutes

Ingredients:

    4 hot dogs

    1 can baked beans

Preparation Instructions: Pre-heat the oven to 375°F. Place the hot dogs on a baking sheet and bake for 10 minutes, until cooked through. Meanwhile, heat the baked beans in a medium saucepan over medium heat. Serve the hot dogs with the baked beans.

9. Sloppy Joes

Prep Time: 15 minutes

Ingredients:

    1 tablespoon oil

    1 cup diced onion

1/2 cup diced bell pepper

1 pound ground beef

1/2 cup ketchup

2 tablespoons Worcestershire sauce

2 tablespoons mustard

Preparation Instructions: Heat the oil in a large skillet over medium heat. Add the onion and bell pepper and cook for 3-4 minutes, until softened. Add the ground beef and cook for 5 minutes, breaking it up with a spoon, until browned. Next is to stir in the ketchup, Worcestershire sauce, and mustard. Simmer for 5 minutes, until the mixture is thickened. Serve it on hamburger buns.

10. Cheesy Broccoli Bites

Prep Time: 15 minutes

Ingredients:

1 package frozen broccoli florets

1 cup shredded cheddar cheese

1/2 cup Italian-style bread crumbs

2 eggs, 2 tablespoons olive oil

Preparation Instructions: Preheat the oven to 375°F.

Place the frozen broccoli florets on a baking sheet and bake for 10 minutes, until softened. Thereafter, allow it to cool a little after removing from the oven. In a shallow bowl, mix together the cheese and bread crumbs. In a separate shallow bowl, beat the eggs. Dip each broccoli floret into the egg, then into the cheese mixture. Then, place the coated florets on the baking sheet. Drizzle with olive oil. Bake for 10-15 minutes, until golden brown and crispy. Serve.

SNACK RECIPES

1. Banana Almond Butter Popcorn

Prep time: 5 minutes

Ingredients:

    4 cups of air-popped popcorn

    2 tablespoons of almond butter

    2 tablespoons of nutella

    2 bananas

    1 teaspoon of cinnamon

Preparation Instructions: Place the popcorn in a large bowl. Heat the almond butter and nutella in a small saucepan over low heat until melted. Cut the bananas into small pieces and add them to the saucepan. Stir in the cinnamon and mix until everything is combined. Pour the mixture over the popcorn and stir until all of the popcorn is coated. Serve and enjoy.

2. Veggie Dip & Crackers

Prep time: 10 minutes

Ingredients:
- 1 cup of plain yogurt
- 1/2 cup of diced cucumber
- 1/2 cup of diced tomatoes
- 1/4 cup of diced peppers
- 2 tablespoons of chopped chives
- 2 tablespoons of olive oil
- 1 teaspoon of garlic powder
- 1 teaspoon of onion powder
- 1 teaspoon of oregano
- 1 package of crackers

Preparation Instructions: Combine the yogurt, cucumber, tomatoes, peppers, and chives in a medium bowl. Add the olive oil, garlic powder, onion powder, and oregano and stir until everything is well combined. Serve the dip with the crackers and enjoy.

3. Chocolate PB & J Smoothie

Prep time: 5 minutes

Ingredients:

    1/2 cup of almond milk

    1/2 cup of frozen strawberries

    1/4 cup of peanut butter

    1 banana

    1 tablespoon of cocoa powder

Preparation Instructions: Place all of the ingredients in a blender and blend until smooth. Serve and enjoy.

4. Trail Mix

Prep time: 5 minutes

Ingredients:

    1/2 cup of almonds

    1/2 cup of walnuts

    1/4 cup of dried cranberries

    1/4 cup of raisins

    1/4 cup of sunflower seeds

Preparation Instructions: Place all of the ingredients in a clean bowl and mix properly until everything is fitly combined. Serve and enjoy.

5. Apple & Cheese Quesadilla

Prep time: 10 minutes

Ingredients:

    2 whole wheat tortillas

    1/2 cup of shredded cheddar cheese

    1/2 cup of diced apples

    2 tablespoons of honey

Preparation Instructions: Pre-heat a skillet over medium heat. Place one of the tortillas in the skillet and sprinkle the cheese, apples, and honey over it. Press down after placing the other tortilla on top. Cook for 3 to 4 minutes, or until the cheese is melted and the tortilla is golden brown. Cut into wedges and serve.

6. Greek Yogurt Parfait

Prep time: 5 minutes

Ingredients:

    1 cup of plain Greek yogurt

1/2 cup of granola

1/2 cup of diced strawberries

Preparation Instructions: Layer the yogurt, granola, and strawberries in a bowl. Serve and enjoy.

7. Frozen Yogurt Bites

Prep time: 10 minutes

Ingredients:

1/2 cup of plain Greek yogurt

1/4 cup of honey

1 teaspoon of vanilla extract

1 cup of fresh berries

Preparation Instructions: Place the yogurt, honey, and vanilla extract in a bowl and mix until everything is combined. Place the berries in a blender and blend until smooth. Add the berry puree to the yogurt mixture and mix until everything is combined. Line a baking sheet with parchment paper and spoon the mixture onto the sheet. Place the baking sheet in the freezer and freeze until the bites are firm. Serve and enjoy.

8. Cucumber & Hummus Snack Pack

Prep time: 5 minutes

Ingredients:

    1 cucumber,

    1/2 cup of hummus

Preparation Instructions: Cut the cucumber into slices. Place the cucumber slices in a container and top with the hummus. Serve and enjoy.

9. Fruit Salad

Prep time: 10 minutes

Ingredients:

    1 cup of diced apples

    1 cup of diced strawberries

    1 cup of diced oranges

    2 tablespoons of honey

Preparation Instructions: Place all of the ingredients in a bowl and mix until everything is combined. Drizzle the honey over the top and mix again. Serve and enjoy.

10. Banana & Peanut Butter Wraps

Prep time: 5 minutes

Ingredients:

2 whole wheat tortillas

2 tablespoons of peanut butter

1 banana

1 teaspoon of cinnamon

Preparation Instructions: Spread the peanut butter over each tortilla. Slice the banana into thin slices and place them on top of the peanut butter. Sprinkle the cinnamon over the top. Roll up the wraps and cut into slices. Serve and enjoy.

DESSERT RECIPES

1. No-Bake Chocolate Oatmeal Cookies

Prep Time: 15 minutes

Ingredients:

    3 tablespoons of butter

    2 tablespoons of honey

    2 tablespoons of cocoa powder

    3 tablespoons of peanut butter

    1/2 cup of oatmeal

    1/4 cup of chocolate chips

Preparation Instructions: Melt the butter in a microwave-safe bowl. Add the honey and cocoa powder and mix together until smooth. Stir in the peanut butter and oatmeal until combined. Line a baking sheet with parchment paper and spoon the mixture into 12 small circles. Place the chocolate chips on top of the mixture and freeze for 15 minutes.)

2. Healthy Fruit Popsicles

Prep Time: 10 minutes

Ingredients:
- 1 cup of fresh strawberries
- 1/2 cup of fresh blueberries
- 1/4 cup of plain Greek yogurt
- 1 tablespoon of honey

Preparation Instructions: Place all the ingredients in a blender and blend thoroughly until very smooth. Pour the mixture into Popsicle molds and freeze for at least 4 hours.

3. Cinnamon Apple Crisp

Prep Time: 25 minutes

Ingredients:

    4 cups of thinly sliced apples

    1/4 cup of brown sugar

    1/4 cup of all-purpose flour

    1/4 cup of rolled oats

    2 tablespoons of butter

    1 teaspoon of ground cinnamon

Preparation Instructions: Pre-heat the oven to 350°F. Grease a 9-inch baking dish and spread the apple slices evenly in the dish. In a separate bowl, combine the brown sugar, flour, oats, butter, and cinnamon and mix until crumbly. Sprinkle the mixture over the apples and bake for 25 minutes or until the apples are tender.

4. Banana Split Pudding Cups

Prep Time: 10 minutes

Ingredients:

    2 ripe bananas

    2 tablespoons of honey

    1 teaspoon of vanilla extract

    2 cups of plain Greek yogurt

    3 tablespoons of mini chocolate chips

1/4 cup of chopped walnuts

Preparation Instructions: Mash the bananas in a bowl and add the honey and vanilla extract. Mix until combined. In 4 small cups, scoop 1/2 cup of yogurt into each cup. Top with the banana mixture, chocolate chips, and walnuts. Refrigerate for at least 1 hour before serving.

5. Baked Apple Chips

Prep Time: 25 minutes

Ingredients:

    2 large apples

    1/4 teaspoon of ground cinnamon

    1/4 teaspoon of nutmeg

Preparation Instructions: Preheat the oven to 200°F. Line a baking sheet with parchment paper. Cut the apples into thin slices and place them on the baking sheet. Sprinkle the cinnamon and nutmeg over the apples. Bake for 25 minutes (or until the apples are crispy). Let them cool before serving.

6. Strawberry-Banana Smoothie

Prep Time: 5 minutes

Ingredients:

- 1/2 cup of plain Greek yogurt
- 1/2 cup of frozen strawberries
- 1/2 banana
- 1/2 cup of almond milk

Preparation Instructions: Place all the ingredients in a blender and blend until smooth. Pour into a glass and enjoy!

7. Frozen Yogurt Bark

Prep Time: 10 minutes

Ingredients:

- 2 cups of plain Greek yogurt
- 1/4 cup of honey
- 1 teaspoon of vanilla extract
- 1/2 cup of chopped almonds
- 1/2 cup of fresh blueberries

Preparation Instructions: Line a baking sheet with parchment paper. In a bowl, combine the yogurt, honey, and vanilla extract and mix until smooth. Spread the mixture onto the parchment paper and sprinkle the almonds and blueberries on top. Freeze for 10 minutes or until solid. Break into pieces and enjoy!

8. Chocolate Banana Bites

Prep Time: 10 minutes

Ingredients:

    1/4 cup of melted semi-sweet chocolate chips

    2 tablespoons of peanut butter

    1 banana

Preparation Instructions: Cut the banana into 1-inch slices and spread the peanut butter on one side of each slice. Place the slices on a parchment-lined baking sheet and drizzle the melted chocolate over them. Place the baking sheet in the freezer for at least 10 minutes before serving.

9. Orange Cake

Prep Time: 30 minutes

Ingredients:

    1/4 cup of butter

    1/4 cup of sugar

    2 eggs

1/4 teaspoon of baking powder

1/2 cup of all-purpose flour

1/2 cup of orange juice

1 teaspoon of orange zest

Preparation Instructions: Preheat the oven to 350°F. Grease a 9-inch round cake pan and set aside. In a large bowl, cream the butter and sugar together. Add the eggs one at a time and mix until combined. In a separate bowl, combine the baking powder and flour and mix together. Slowly add the flour mixture to the butter mixture and mix until combined. Add the orange juice and zest and mix until combined. Pour the mixture into the prepared cake pan and bake for 30 minutes or until a toothpick inserted in the center comes out clean.

10. Rice Crispy Treats

Prep Time: 15 minutes

Ingredients:

3 tablespoons of butter

4 cups of mini marshmallows

6 cups of crisp rice cereal

Preparation Instructions: Grease a 9x13 baking dish

with butter. Melt the butter over medium heat in a large pan. Stir rigorously until completely melted while adding the marshmallows. Remove the pan from the heat and stir in the cereal. Press the mixture into the prepared baking dish and let cool for 15 minutes before cutting into bars.

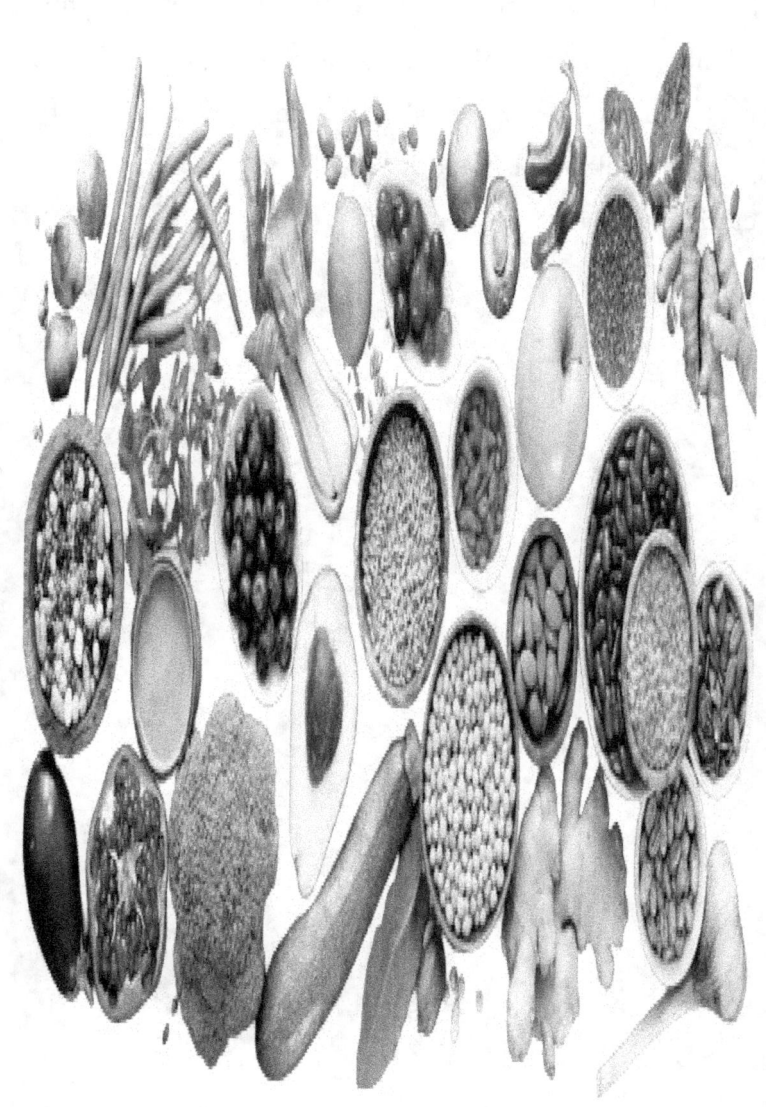

CHAPTER 5

MEAL PLANNING

Meal planning for kids with cancer can be a daunting task. It is important to provide meals that are not only nutritious but also easy to prepare and tasty. Here are some tips to help make meal planning easier and more effective for kids with cancer:

1. Make sure to include plenty of fruits and vegetables in your meal planning. Fruits and vegetables are packed with vitamins, minerals, and other nutrients that can help boost the immune system and provide energy. Incorporate a variety of colors and textures to make meals more enjoyable.

2. Include healthy proteins such as lean meats, nuts, legumes, and eggs. Protein helps to maintain muscle mass and strength, which is important for kids with cancer.

3. Try to limit unhealthy fats and processed foods. Fried foods and high-fat snacks can increase the risk of weight gain and other health issues.

4. Incorporate healthy snacks throughout the day. This can help to provide extra energy and nutrition for kids with cancer. Healthy snacks such as yogurt, nuts, and fruits are great options.

5. Don't be afraid to get creative with meal planning. Incorporate recipes that are both healthy and fun. Try to involve the kids in the meal planning process to make it more enjoyable.

6. Make sure to include a variety of flavors and textures. This will help to keep meals interesting and enjoyable.

7. Ensure to get adequate rest and sleep. Eating a balanced diet is important, but so is getting enough rest. Make sure to include plenty of rest in your meal planning.

Meal planning for kids with cancer can be challenging.

By following these tips, you can help make meal planning easier and more effective for your child. With a little bit of creativity and planning, you can provide your child with delicious, nutritious meals that will help to keep them healthy and energized. Below is a 7 day kid-friendly meal plan you can try out for kids with cancer.

DAY 1

BREAKFAST: Overnight oats made with almond milk, chia seeds, and fresh blueberries

Prep Time: 10 minutes

Ingredients:
- -1/2 cup old-fashioned oats
- -1/2 cup almond milk
- -2 tablespoons chia seeds
- -1/4 cup fresh blueberries
- -1 teaspoon honey (optional)

Preparation Instructions:

1. In a medium-sized bowl, combine the oats, almond milk, and chia seeds. Stir until the ingredients are well-combined.

2. Add the blueberries and stir until evenly distributed.

3. Cover the bowl with plastic wrap or a lid and place in the refrigerator overnight.

4. In the morning, remove the bowl from the refrigerator and add honey, if desired. Serve chilled.

LUNCH: Quinoa and black bean salad with grilled vegetables

Prep Time: 15 minutes

Ingredients:
- 1 cup of quinoa
- 1 can of rinsed and drained black beans
- 1 bell pepper, chopped
- 1 red onion, chopped
- 1 zucchini, chopped
- Freshly squeezed lime juice, 1/4 cup
- 2 tablespoons of olive oil
- 1 tablespoon of garlic, minced
- 1 teaspoon of cumin
- 1 teaspoon of chili powder
- 1/2 teaspoon of sea salt
- 1/4 teaspoon of black pepper
- 1/4 cup of cilantro, chopped

Preparation Instructions:

1. To prepare the quinoa, follow the directions on the box.
2. In a large bowl, combine the cooked quinoa, black beans, bell pepper, red onion, and zucchini.
3. In a separate bowl, whisk together the lime juice, olive oil, garlic, cumin, chili powder, salt, and pepper.
4. Pour the dressing over the quinoa mixture and stir to combine.
5. Heat a large skillet over medium-high heat and add the vegetables.
6. Grill the vegetables for about 5 minutes or until they are tender and lightly charred.
7. Add the grilled vegetables to the quinoa mixture and stir to combine.
8. Top with cilantro and serve. Enjoy!

DINNER: Baked salmon filet with roasted potatoes and a side salad

Prep Time: 15 minutes
Cook Time: 35 minutes

Ingredients:

- 2 salmon filets
- 2 tablespoons olive oil
- 2 cloves garlic, minced
- 2 teaspoons dried oregano
- 2 teaspoons paprika
- 2 teaspoons lemon juice
- 2 tablespoons butter
- 1 pound baby potatoes, halved
- Salt and pepper, to taste
- 2 tablespoons chopped fresh parsley
- 4 cups mixed greens
- 2 tablespoons balsamic vinaigrette

Preparation Instructions:

1. Preheat the oven to 400°F.
2. Salmon filets should be put on a baking dish. Drizzle with olive oil and sprinkle with garlic, oregano, paprika, lemon juice, salt, and pepper. top with butter.
3. Place the potatoes in a separate baking dish. Olive oil should be drizzled and salt and pepper should be sprinkled.
4. Bake both dishes for 25–30 minutes, or until the

potatoes are tender and the salmon is cooked through.

5. Meanwhile, in a large bowl, combine mixed greens and balsamic vinaigrette. Greens should be covered uniformly after mixing.

6. To serve, divide the salad among plates. Top each plate with a salmon filet and potatoes. Sprinkle with parsley. Enjoy!

DAY 2

BREAKFAST: Scrambled eggs with spinach and tomatoes

Prep Time: 10 minutes

Ingredients:
- 4 eggs
- 2 tablespoons of butter or oil
- ½ cup of fresh spinach
- ½ cup of chopped tomatoes
- Salt and pepper to taste

Preparation Instructions:

1. Crack the eggs into a bowl and whisk together until combined.

2. Heat the butter or oil over medium heat in a skillet.

3. Add the spinach and tomatoes to the skillet and sauté for a few minutes until cooked through.

4. Add the eggs to the skillet and stir continuously until the eggs are cooked to desired consistency.

5. Add salt and pepper to taste.

6. Serve the scrambled eggs with spinach and tomatoes and enjoy!

LUNCH: Lentil soup with a side of crackers

Prep Time: 20 minutes

Ingredients:
- 2 tablespoons olive oil
- 1 onion, diced
- 2 cloves garlic, minced
- 2 carrots, diced
- 2 stalks celery, diced
- 2 cups washed and dried green or brown lentils
- 6 cups vegetable broth
- 2 bay leaves
- 1 teaspoon cumin
- Salt and pepper, to taste

- Crackers, for serving

Preparation Instructions:

1. In a big saucepan, heat the olive oil on medium-high.
2. Add the onion, garlic, carrots, and celery to the pot and cook until the vegetables are softened, about 5 minutes.
3. Add the lentils, vegetable broth, bay leaves, and cumin to the pot and bring to a boil.
4. Reduce the heat and simmer until the lentils are tender, about 15 minutes.
5. After removing the bay leaves, season to taste with salt and pepper.
6. Serve the soup warm with crackers. Enjoy!

DINNER: Baked chicken breast with mashed sweet potatoes and roasted Brussels sprouts

Prep Time: 30 minutes

Ingredients:

- 4 boneless, skinless chicken breasts
- 2 tablespoons of olive oil
- 2 tablespoons of garlic powder
- 2 tablespoons of onion powder

- 2 tablespoons of paprika
- 2 tablespoons of dried oregano
- Salt and pepper to taste
- 2 cups of mashed sweet potatoes
- 1 cup of Brussels sprouts
- 2 tablespoons of olive oil
- 2 tablespoons of garlic powder
- 2 tablespoons of onion powder
- 2 tablespoons of paprika
- 2 tablespoons of dried oregano
- Salt and pepper to taste

Preparation Instructions:

1. Preheat the oven to 375°F.

2. In a small bowl, combine the olive oil, garlic powder, onion powder, paprika, oregano, salt, and pepper.

3. Rub the chicken breasts with the spice mixture and place them on a baking sheet lined with parchment paper.

4. Bake the chicken for 25–30 minutes, until it is cooked through.

5. Meanwhile, in a small bowl, combine the mashed sweet potatoes, Brussels sprouts, olive oil, garlic

powder, onion powder, paprika, oregano, salt, and pepper.

6. Place the mixture on a baking sheet lined with parchment paper and bake for 20 minutes until the vegetables are tender.

7. Serve the chicken with the mashed sweet potatoes and roasted Brussels sprouts. Enjoy!

DAY 3

BREAKFAST: Oat and banana pancakes

Prep Time: 10 minutes

Ingredients:
- 2 cups rolled oats
- 2 ripe bananas
- 2 eggs
- 1 teaspoon baking powder
- ½ teaspoon ground cinnamon
- 2 tablespoons honey
- 2 tablespoons olive oil
- 1 cup almond milk
- 1 teaspoon vanilla extract

- Pinch of salt

Preparation Instructions:

1. In a blender, add the rolled oats, bananas, eggs, baking powder, cinnamon, honey, olive oil, almond milk, vanilla extract and salt. Blend until smooth.
2. Heat a non-stick skillet over medium heat and add a tablespoon of olive oil.
3. Pour ¼ cup of the batter into the skillet and spread evenly.
4. Cook for 2-3 minutes on each side or until golden brown.
5. Repeat with the remaining batter.
6. Serve the pancakes with your favorite toppings, such as maple syrup, fresh fruit, or nut butter. Enjoy!

LUNCH: Hummus wrap with mixed greens, tomatoes, and cucumbers

Prep Time: 15 minutes

Ingredients:

- 2 large whole wheat wraps
- 2 tablespoons of hummus
- 2 cups of mixed greens

- 2 Roma tomatoes, diced
- 1 cucumber, diced
- 2 tablespoons of olive oil
- Salt and pepper to taste

Preparation Instructions:

1. A big skillet should be placed at minimal heat.
2. Spread one tablespoon of hummus onto each wrap.
3. Add mixed greens, tomatoes, and cucumbers to the wraps and season with salt and pepper.
4. Drizzle the wraps with olive oil and fold them up.
5. Place the wraps in the heated skillet and cook until golden brown and crispy, flipping once.
6. Serve the hummus wrap with mixed greens, tomatoes, and cucumbers warm and enjoy!

DINNER: Baked tilapia with brown rice and steamed broccoli

Prep Time: 15 minutes

Ingredients:

- 2 tilapia fillets
- 2 cups cooked brown rice
- 2 cups steamed broccoli

- 2 tablespoons olive oil
- 1 teaspoon garlic powder
- 1 teaspoon Italian seasoning
- 1 teaspoon paprika
- Salt and pepper to taste

Preparation Instructions:

1. Preheat oven to 375°F.
2. Place tilapia fillets in a baking dish.
3. Drizzle with olive oil and sprinkle with garlic powder, Italian seasoning, paprika, salt, and pepper.
4. Bake for 15 minutes.
5. Divide cooked brown rice and steamed broccoli between two plates.
6. Top each plate with a tilapia fillet.
7. Enjoy!

DAY 4

BREAKFAST: Smoothie bowl made with almond milk, banana, and frozen berries

Prep Time: 5 minutes

Ingredients:

- 1 cup almond milk
- 1 banana
- 1/2 cup frozen berries (such as blueberries, raspberries, blackberries, etc.)
- Toppings (optional): chia seeds, shredded coconut, nuts, etc.

Preparation Instructions:

1. In a blender, add almond milk, bananas, and frozen berries.
2. Blend rigorously until it becomes very smooth
3. Pour the smoothie into a bowl.
4. Add desired toppings and mix.
5. Enjoy your smoothie bowl!

LUNCH: Kale and quinoa salad with a side of carrots and hummus

Prep time: 15 minutes

Ingredients:

- 2 cups of cooked quinoa
- 2 cups of kale, chopped
- 2 tablespoons of olive oil
- 2 cloves of garlic, minced

- Salt and pepper, to taste
- 2 carrots cut into thin slices
- 2 tablespoons of tahini
- 2 tablespoons of lemon juice
- 2 tablespoons of water
- 2 tablespoons of olive oil

Preparation Instructions:

1. In a large mixing bowl, combine the cooked quinoa and chopped kale.

2. In a separate small bowl, mix together the olive oil, garlic, salt, and pepper.

3. Pour the oil mixture over the quinoa and kale and stir to combine.

4. Place the quinoa and kale mixture in a large skillet over medium heat. Cook for about five minutes, and stir once in a while.

5. Meanwhile, prepare the hummus. In a small bowl, mix together the tahini, lemon juice, water, and olive oil.

6. Add the carrot slices to the skillet and cook for an additional 5 minutes.

7. Serve the quinoa and kale mixture with the hummus and carrots. Enjoy!

DINNER: Grilled tofu with roasted vegetables and a side of brown rice

Prep Time: 15 minutes
Cook Time: 30 minutes
Total Time: 45 minutes
Servings: 4
Ingredients:
- 1 package of extra-firm tofu, cut into cubes
- 1 red bell pepper, thinly sliced
- 1 yellow bell pepper, thinly sliced
- 1 orange bell pepper, thinly sliced
- One red onion, thinly sliced
- 2 tablespoons olive oil
- 2 teaspoons smoked paprika
- 1 teaspoon garlic powder
- 1 teaspoon sea salt
- 1 teaspoon black pepper
- 2 cups cooked brown rice

Preparation Instructions:
1. Preheat your grill to medium-high heat.
2. In a large bowl, add the tofu cubes and bell peppers. Drizzle the olive oil over the top and mix until

everything is evenly coated.

3. In a small bowl, mix together the smoked paprika, garlic powder, sea salt and black pepper. Sprinkle the seasoning over the tofu and vegetables and mix until everything is evenly coated.

4. Place the tofu and vegetables on the preheated grill. Grill for 15 minutes, flipping the tofu and vegetables halfway through.

5. While the tofu and vegetables are grilling, cook the brown rice according to package instructions.

6. Serve the grilled tofu and vegetables over a bed of brown rice. Enjoy!

DAY 5

BREAKFAST: Oatmeal with almond butter and raisins

Prep Time: 5 minutes

Ingredients:
- -1 cup of rolled oats
- -1 cup of almond milk
- -1 tablespoon of almond butter

- 2 tablespoons of raisins
- 1 tablespoon of honey
- 1 teaspoon of ground cinnamon
- 1/4 teaspoon of salt

Preparation Instructions:

1. In a medium saucepan, bring almond milk to a boil over medium-high heat.
2. Add in the rolled oats and reduce the heat to low.
3. Stir the oats until they have absorbed the milk, about two minutes.
4. Remove the pan from the heat and stir in almond butter, raisins, honey, cinnamon, and salt.
5. Serve the oatmeal warm, topped with a drizzle of honey and extra raisins if desired. Enjoy!

LUNCH: Spinach and avocado sandwich with a side of fruit

Prep Time: 10 minutes

Ingredients:
- 2 slices of sandwich bread
- 1/4 cup of spinach leaves
- 1/4 of a ripe avocado, sliced

- 1 tablespoon of mayonnaise
- 1 teaspoon of lemon juice
- 1/4 teaspoon of garlic powder
- Salt & pepper to taste
- Assorted fruit (berries, bananas, oranges, etc.)

Preparation Instructions:

1. Toast the two slices of sandwich bread.

2. In a small bowl, mash the avocado and combine with the mayonnaise, lemon juice, garlic powder, and a pinch of salt and pepper.

3. Spread the avocado mixture onto one slice of the toasted bread.

4. Top the avocado mixture with the spinach leaves.

5. Place the other slice of toasted bread on top of the spinach.

6. Cut the sandwich into halves and serve with a side of assorted fruit. Enjoy!

DINNER: Baked sweet potato with black beans, spinach, and salsa

Prep Time: 15 minutes

Ingredients:

- 2 Sweet Potatoes
- 1 can of black beans
- 1/4 cup of salsa
- 2 cups of spinach
- Salt & Pepper
- Olive Oil

Preparation Instructions:

1. Preheat the oven to 375 °F.
2. Rinse and scrub the sweet potatoes.
3. Pierce the sweet potatoes with a fork and place on a baking sheet. Bake for 40 minutes.
4. Rinse and drain the black beans.
5. Using a small pan, heat the olive oil with a little heat. Add the black beans, spinach, and salsa and sauté for 5 minutes.
6. Once the sweet potatoes have finished baking, cut them in half and top with the black bean mixture.
7. Sprinkle with salt and pepper and serve. Enjoy!

DAY 6

BREAKFAST: Chia seed pudding with fresh

berries

Prep Time: 10 minutes

Ingredients:

-1/4 cup Chia Seeds

-1 cup Coconut Milk

-1/2 teaspoon Vanilla Extract

-2 tablespoons Maple Syrup

-1/4 teaspoon Ground Cinnamon

-Fresh Berries, 1 cup (Strawberries, Blueberries, Raspberries, etc.)

Preparation Instructions:

1. In a medium-sized bowl, whisk together the chia seeds, coconut milk, vanilla extract, maple syrup, and cinnamon until well combined.

2. Transfer the pudding mixture to a storage container or bowl and refrigerate for at least 4 hours or overnight.

3. When the pudding has set, top with fresh berries and serve. Enjoy!

LUNCH: Chickpea and kale salad with a side of mixed nuts

Prep Time: 10 minutes

Ingredients:

- 2 cups cooked chickpeas
- 2 cups chopped kale
- 1 red onion, diced
- 1/4 cup extra-virgin olive oil
- 2 tablespoons white vinegar
- 1 teaspoon dijon mustard
- 1/4 cup fresh parsley, chopped
- 1/2 teaspoon sea salt
- 1/2 teaspoon freshly ground black pepper
- 1/2 cup mixed nuts, such as almonds, walnuts and cashews

Preparation Instructions:

1. In a large bowl, combine chickpeas, kale, and red onion.
2. In a small bowl, whisk together olive oil, vinegar, Dijon mustard, parsley, salt, and pepper to make a dressing.
3. Pour dressing over the chickpea and kale mixture and toss to combine.
4. Serve the salad with a side of mixed nuts. Enjoy!

DINNER: Turkey burger with roasted sweet potatoes and a side of steamed vegetables

Prep Time: 15 minutes

Ingredients:
- 1 pound ground turkey
- 2 tablespoons olive oil
- 1 teaspoon garlic powder
- 1 teaspoon onion powder
- 1 teaspoon smoked paprika
- 1 teaspoon chili powder
- 2 tablespoons Worcestershire sauce
- 2 sweet potatoes, cubed
- 1/2 teaspoon sea salt
- 1/4 teaspoon black pepper
- 2 tablespoons olive oil
- 2 cups of your favorite vegetables (broccoli, carrots, green beans, etc.)

Preparation Instructions:

1. Preheat the oven to 400 °F.
2. In a large bowl, combine the ground turkey, 2 tablespoons of olive oil, garlic powder, onion powder, smoked paprika, chili powder, and Worcestershire

sauce. Form the mixture into 4-6 patties.

3. Place the cubed sweet potatoes on a parchment-lined baking sheet and toss with 2 tablespoons of olive oil, sea salt, and black pepper. Bake for 15-20 minutes, until the potatoes are tender and golden.

4. Heat a large skillet over medium-high heat. Cook the turkey burgers for about 5 minutes per side, or until the internal temperature reaches 165°F.

5. Meanwhile, heat a pot of water over high heat and add the vegetables. The veggies should be soft after 5 minutes of simmering after bringing to a boil.

6. Serve the turkey burgers with roasted sweet potatoes and steamed vegetables. Enjoy!

DAY 7

BREAKFAST: Yogurt parfait with granola and fresh fruit

Prep Time: 10 minutes

Ingredients:
- 1 cup plain Greek yogurt
- 1/4 cup of your favorite granola

- 1/4 cup of fresh blueberries
- 1/4 cup of fresh raspberries
- 1/4 cup of fresh blackberries
- 1 tablespoon of honey
- 1 tablespoon of slivered almonds

Preparation Instructions:

1. In a medium-sized bowl, combine the yogurt and honey. Stir until the yogurt is completely mixed with the honey.
2. Place the granola in a separate bowl.
3. Place the fresh fruit into a third bowl.
4. To assemble the parfait, take a medium-sized glass or cup and spoon in a layer of the yogurt and honey mixture.
5. Top the yogurt with a layer of granola, followed by a layer of fruit.
6. Repeat, layering the yogurt, granola, and fruit until the glass or cup is full.
7. Sprinkle the slivered almonds on top of the parfait.
8. Serve and enjoy!

LUNCH: Veggie wrap with hummus and mixed

greens

Prep Time: 10 minutes

Ingredients:

- 2 whole wheat wraps
- 2 tablespoons of hummus
- 1/4 cup of mixed greens
- 1/4 cup of grated carrots
- 1/4 cup of diced cucumbers
- 1/4 cup of diced tomatoes
- 1/4 cup of diced red onion

Preparation Instructions:

1. Spread the hummus evenly across the two wraps.

2. Place the mixed greens on top of the hummus.

3. Sprinkle the grated carrots, diced cucumbers, diced tomatoes, and diced red onion on top of the mixed greens.

4. Wrap the wrap by folding the sides in and rolling it up.

5. Cut the wrap in half and serve. Enjoy!

DINNER: Baked salmon with quinoa and roasted asparagus

Prep time: 15 minutes
Cook time: 25 minutes
Total time: 40 minutes
Serves: 4
Ingredients:
- 4 salmon fillets (6 ounces each)
- 1 tablespoon olive oil
- Salt and pepper to taste
- 1 cup quinoa
- 2 cups vegetable broth
- 2 cloves garlic, minced
- 1/4 cup freshly squeezed lemon juice
- 1/4 cup freshly chopped parsley
- 1 pound of trimmed and divided into 2-inch pieces asparagus
- 1 tablespoon olive oil
- 2 tablespoons freshly grated Parmesan cheese

Preparation Instructions:

1. Preheat oven to 400 °F.

2. Salmon fillets should be placed on a baking pan covered with parchment paper. Olive oil should be drizzled and salt and pepper should be sprinkled.

Salmon should be baked for 15 to 20 minutes, or until done.

3. Meanwhile, in a medium saucepan, bring quinoa and vegetable broth to a boil. Reduce heat to medium and let the quinoa simmer for fifteen minutes, or until fully cooked.

4. In a small bowl, mix together garlic, lemon juice, and parsley.

5. In a separate bowl, toss asparagus with olive oil, salt, and pepper. Transfer to a baking sheet and bake for 10–15 minutes, or until asparagus is tender and lightly browned.

6. To assemble, divide cooked quinoa among four plates. Top with salmon fillets and asparagus. Drizzle with the lemon garlic parsley mixture and sprinkle with Parmesan cheese. Serve immediately.

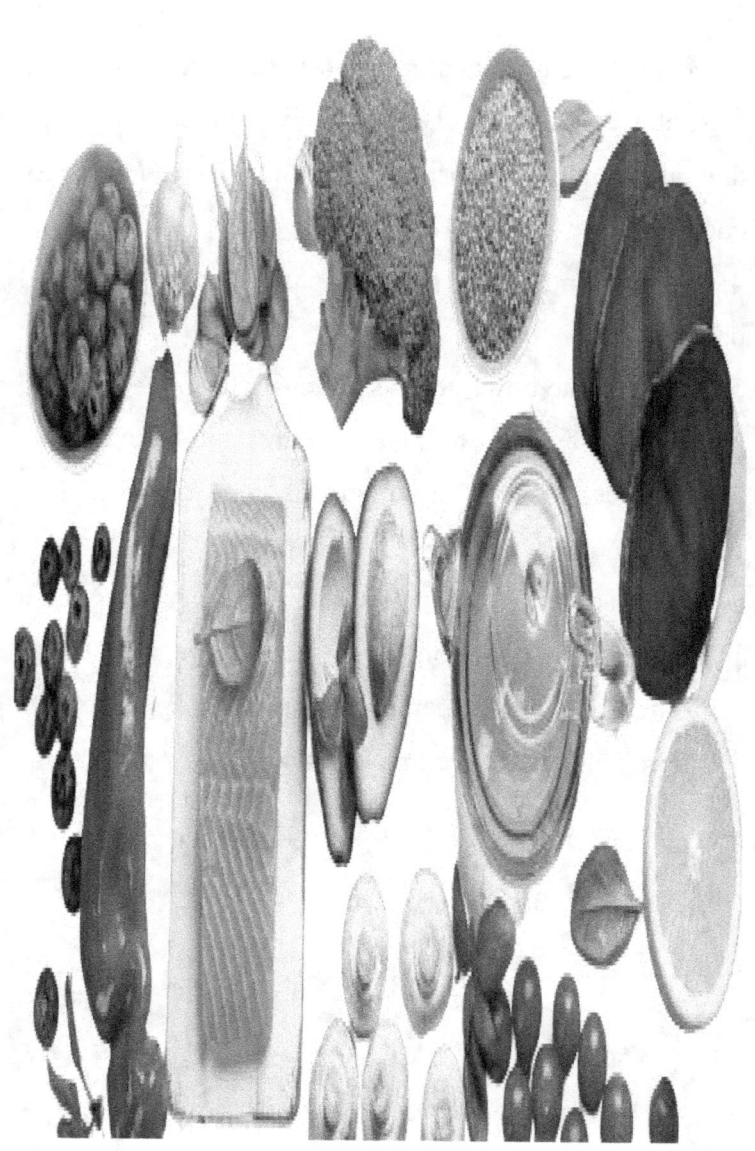

CHAPTER 6

TIPS FOR ENCOURAGING KIDS TO EAT HEALTHY

Eating healthy is essential for good health, especially for children with cancer. But this may be difficult for kids with cancer, who may experience a loss of appetite, nausea, vomiting, or taste changes due to their illness or treatments. Here are a few tips to help encourage kids with cancer to eat healthfully:

1. **Make meals fun:** Make meals interactive and fun by letting the child help with meal preparation, or by adding fun foods like fresh fruits or vegetables to a dish.

2. **Choose nutrient-rich foods:** Choose foods that are high in nutrients, such as lean proteins, fresh fruits and vegetables, and whole grains.

3. **Offer smaller, more frequent meals:** Offer smaller meals throughout the day, rather than three large meals. This will help to keep the child's energy level up and prevent them from feeling overwhelmed.

4. **Stick to a routine:** Eating at the same time every day can help to establish a healthy eating routine.

5. **Offer variety:** Try to offer a variety of foods to keep meals interesting and appealing.

6. **Make snacks available:** Make healthy snacks available throughout the day, such as fresh fruits, vegetables, and nuts. You can as well try out other delicious snack recipes provided in this book.

7. **Offer food rewards:** Offer rewards for eating healthy foods, such as a special activity or movie night.

8. **Get creative:** Get creative with food, such as mixing different flavors or textures together to make interesting

dishes.

9. **Let them decide:** Let the child make decisions about what to eat. This will help them to feel in control and more likely to eat.

10. **Make it accessible:** Make healthy food easily accessible, such as keeping it in plain view or pre-packing it for convenience.

These tips can help to make healthy eating easier and more enjoyable for kids with cancer. Eating healthy can help to keep their bodies strong and give them the energy they need to fight their illness. However, it is also noteworthy for parents, guardians, and love ones to be on the look out for the lifestyle changes that accompany kids diagnosed with cancer. Taking note of these changes coupled with adequate attention will positively affect the overall child's health and response to treatment.

LIFESTYLE CHANGES TO CONSIDER

It is important to be aware of the lifestyle changes that may be necessary for children with cancer. These changes in lifestyle may be necessary to maintain the child's health and well-being.

NUTRITION: A healthy diet is essential for children with cancer. The child's diet should be tailored to the type of cancer they have and the treatments they are receiving. It is important to provide a balanced diet that includes plenty of fruits and vegetables, lean proteins, and whole grains. The child should also be encouraged to drink plenty of fluids and get enough sleep.

ACTIVITY: Regular physical activity is important for children with cancer. Depending on the type of cancer and treatment, the child may need to adjust their activity level. For some children, this may mean increasing their activity level, while for others it may mean limiting their activity. It is important to consult with the child's doctor to determine the appropriate level of activity.

MENTAL HEALTH: Mental health is an important part of the overall health of a child with cancer. It is important to provide emotional support to the child and their family. This can include counseling, support groups, and other forms of therapy.

SOCIALIZATION: Socialization is an important part of a child's life. It is important to provide opportunities for the child to interact with their peers and engage in activities that they enjoy. This can help them stay positive and connected to their peers.

MEDICAL MANAGEMENT: Proper medical management is important for any child with cancer. The child's doctor should be consulted to determine the best course of treatment. This may include medications, surgery, radiation, or chemotherapy. It is also important to follow up on any tests or other procedures that the doctor orders.

These are some of the lifestyle changes that may be necessary for a child with cancer. It is important to consult with the child's doctor to determine the best course of action for the child. It is also important to provide support and encouragement to the child and their family throughout this difficult time.

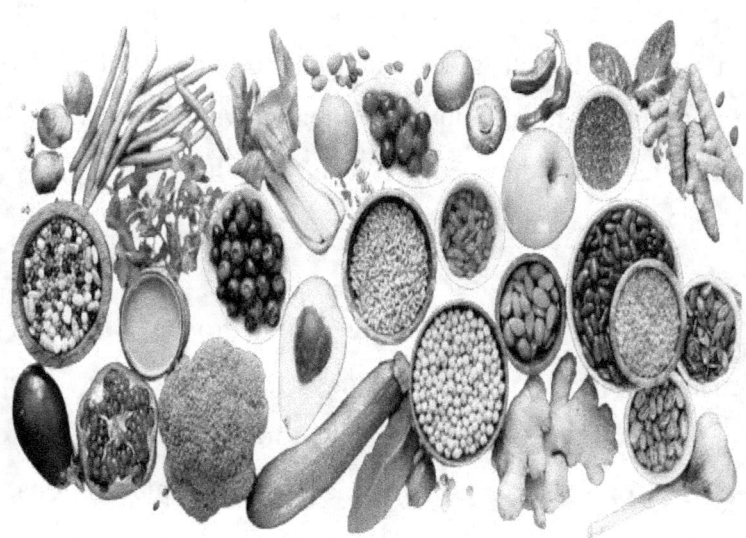

CONCLUSION

We have discussed various cancer diet recipes for kids, from easy-to-prepare meals to more elaborate dishes. These recipes are designed to help kids get the most out of their meals and keep them healthy.

By providing a wide variety of healthy and delicious options, kids can find recipes that appeal to them and their families. They can enjoy meals that are both nutritious and tasty. Additionally, the recipes are designed to provide the necessary vitamins and minerals that are important for healthy growth and development.

Making sure that kids get the right nutrients is important for their overall well-being. With cancer diet recipes for kids, parents can rest assured that their children are getting the best nutrition possible, as well as having fun while doing it. With a variety of recipes to choose from, kids can find something that they enjoy and that is beneficial for their healt

www.ingramcontent.com/pod-product-compliance
Lightning Source LLC
Chambersburg PA
CBHW070252220526
45465CB00004B/1597